Being Fabulously Fit In God's Kingdom

A 40-Day Journey to Wellness

Renee Wiggins

Being Fabulously Fit: A 40-Day Journey to Wellness

© 2013 by Renee Wiggins

ISBN: 978-0-9825613-3-1

First printing

This book was printed in the United States of America.

Scripture quotations marked (AMP) are taken from the **Amplified Bible**. Copyright © 1954, 1958, 1962, 1964, 1965, 1987 by The Lockman Foundation. Used by permission.

Scripture marked (MSG) are taken from The Message. Copyright © 1993, 1994, 1995, 1996, 2000, 2001, 2002. Used by permission of NavPress Publishing Group.

Scripture quotations marked (NIV) are taken from the Holy Bible, New International Version®, NIV®. Copyright © 1973, 1978, 1984, 2011 by Biblica, Inc.™ Used by permission of Zondervan. All rights reserved worldwide. www.zondervan.com.

The "NIV" and "New International Version" are trademarks registered in the United States Patent and Trademark Office by Biblica, Inc.™

Scripture quotations marked (NKJV) are taken from the New King James Version®. Copyright © 1982 by Thomas Nelson, Inc. Used by permission. All rights reserved.

Scripture quotations marked (TNIV) are taken from the Holy Bible, Today's New International Version®. Copyright © 2001, 2005 by Biblica®. Used by permission of Biblica®. All rights reserved worldwide.

"TNIV" and "Today's New International Version" are trademarks registered in the United States Patent and Trademark Office by Biblica®. Use of either trademark requires the permission of Biblica.

To order additional copies of this book, contact:
Results By Renee
www.resultsbyrenee.com

Cover design by Tyora Twebbin of http://tywebbincreations.com/

Page layout by Jera Publishing of http://www.self-pub.net/

The exercises described in this book are from established exercise programs, but they are not a substitute for medical advice given by a physician. Always consult your physician first before starting any exercise program. If you should start feeling faint, dizzy, or have physical discomfort, you should stop immediately and consult your physician.

The purpose of this book is solely to educate, and it is sold with the understanding that the author and the publisher are neither liable nor responsible for any injury alleged to be caused directly or indirectly by the information in this book.

Dedication

To my parents, sisters, nieces, colleagues, and clients for all your support and encouragement.

Acknowledgments

Thanks to all my friends, colleagues, and clients who have shaped and supported and encouraged me to go beyond.

Thanks to Tyora Tywebbin of Tywebbin Creations, who helped me develop this book.

Thanks to my editor, my friend Kathy Grow, for helping shape this book for final publication. You always asked the right questions.

Thanks to Reggi Johnson- for helping me to develop the "Know Your Numbers for Spiritual Fitness."

Thanks to Sheila Johnson for helping me to develop the " The Last Supper " pages.

Praise For
Being Fabulously Fit
In God's Kingdom

Renee Wiggins has created a 40-day journey that will certainly benefit the Body of Christ. *Being Fabulously Fit in God's Kingdom* expertly combines the physical with the spiritual to achieve the goal of total wellness—which is God's plan for His children.

Kara Davis, M.D.
Physician and Author
Spiritual Secrets to Weight Loss
Spiritual Secrets to a Healthy Heart

If you are serious about taking care of yourself then I highly recommend Being Fabulously Fit in God's Kingdom. Renee takes the reader on a 40-day journey offering practical and spiritual tips to achieve greater fitness from the inside out.

Janet G. Daughtry, M.DIV, CBC, LBC
Co-Founder of Life Breakthrough Academy
Life and Leadership Breakthrough Coach
Transforming Lives Through Coaching and Coach Training

This is a very thoughtful, Spirit-inspired approach to meditation and contemplation to motivate us to a healthier lifestyle. Renee's suggestions are practical, accurate and build upon themselves in a manner that as the 40 days go by, you could be "resurrected" to a new, healthier you! Thank you for representing nutrition and health from a sensible, scriptural perspective that isn't a prescription for taking supplements and pills, but instead, coaches a change from the inside-out!

Terry Lykins, RD
Author of *Soul Food:
A Dietitian' s Guide to Nutritional Transformation*

You must maximize your body to maximize your impact for God. Being Fabulously Fit In God's Kingdom is a great resource for making this happen. It is packed with information that can help you create and maintain a healthy lifestyle. God will be honored and your body with thank you for taking 40 days to read and apply this book.

Steve Reynolds
Senior Pastor, Capital Baptist Church, Annandale, VA
Author of *Bod4God* and *Get Off The Couch*

Contents

To the Reader:
The Journey

[19] Do you not know that your bodies are temples of the Holy Spirit, who is in you, whom you have received from God? You are not your own; [20] you were bought at a price. Therefore honor God with your bodies.

1 Corinthians 6:19-21 (NIV)

God has given each of us our first breath. He lives inside of us. Yet, we have abused our bodies/temples.

How? By overeating, lack of sleep, and lack of physical exercise, all needed to keep our temples strong. In addition, we take on too much and that eventually wears us down.

God gives us what we can handle, but we do not listen to him and we pay for it. We pay with uncontrollable high blood pressure, stress, obesity, and bone and joint diseases.

If we truly believe God lives in us, then we will not abuse our bodies, but honor them with the proper nourishment, exercise, and love.

We tend to our cars and beautify our homes, but spend much less time, money, and effort on taking care of ourselves.

By picking up this book, you have committed yourself toward getting healthy by living God's Word.

This book is for YOU. It is to be used as part of your journey in life.

Introduction

Mirror, Mirror, who is the fairest of them all? Mirror, Mirror, who is the most Fit and Fabulous of them all?

It is you. God created you in his image. Look into the mirror and know you are *somebody* and you have the power. Beauty begins within, and most women do not realize how beautiful they are and how fit they are.

As young adults, we took health for granted. The temples God gave us endured sleepless nights, overeating, drinking, smoking, and drugs.

But health is a gift from God, and our bodies should be nourished, respected, loved, and taken care of—each and every day.

God lives in us and we live in him. Honor and obey.

The keys to keeping the body healthy are exercise and eating right. We must also flex our spiritual muscles, by practicing prayer and meditation and by reading the Word.

Physical fitness provides us with flexibility, endurance, strength, and power to do daily activities. Balancing physical health with the spiritual can strengthen the mind, body, and soul.

To be a Fit and Fabulous Woman of God, one must seek God's Word first when making healthy choices. Love yourself first, so others will also love you.

Fit and Fabulous Women of God: we do not live by bread alone, but also with the Word. Cherish, honor, nourish, and love this gift from God—your body.

Prayer:

Thanks, God, for creating me. I will treat this body with care and love. Thanks for these blessings.

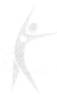

DAY 1

God's Image vs. Our Image

Scripture

[14] *I will confess and praise You for You are fearful and wonderful and for the awful wonder of my birth! Wonderful are Your works, and that my inner self knows right well.*

PSALM 139:14 (AMP)

Devotional

We were created in God's image. He doesn't make any mistakes or failures, yet we disrespect him by rejecting what God has made. God molded—shaped—us with clay and mud to form his likeness and to serve him.

Yet millions of Americans are not happy with their bodies. They choose to go on diets that don't work, or some choose to have surgery to remove this or fix that. And, after it is all done, they are still not happy.

Yes, you can have plastic surgery or lose a lot of weight using liquids or pills, but are you truly happy with yourself?

Happiness—a feeling of self-worth—begins inside, not outside. As a Life Coach, I help women tap the powers they have within, so they find the solutions for themselves.

And those solutions begin on the inside and work their way to the outside.

Prayer

Dear Heavenly Father, encourage me to accept who I am. After all, I was made in your image and you do not make any mistakes.

Questions

Do you find yourself comparing yourself to others?

☐ Yes ☐ No

If Yes, why?

_____

_____

_____

You were made in God's image, not man's image. Be happy about your body and looks.

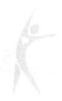

DAY 2
Prayer Knocks Down Walls

Scripture

17. . . [P]ray continually, 18 give thanks in all circumstances; for this is God's will for you in Christ Jesus. 19 Do not quench the Spirit.

1 THESSALONIANS 5:17-19 (NIV)

Devotional

Prayer heals all things. Prayer conquers all things, too.

I used to love eating chocolate chip cookies. When payday came along, I would go and buy Mrs. Fields™ Chocolate Chip Cookies. They would melt in my mouth. I didn't care about the price or how far I had to travel to get them.

Until one day, when I noticed the price had almost doubled. What? Ninety-eight cents for one cookie? "No way," I said.

However, the urge was still very strong until I simply had to pray for God to take the craving away from me. I prayed long and hard.

I knew praying had worked for me the day I went to the local mall and walked right past the cookies. My sister and nieces were surprised!

If you have a hard time losing weight or staying with your exercise plan, ask for God to give you the strength to stay on track.

Prayer

Dear Heavenly Father, I am afraid I might lose the battle. Hold my hand. *Teach me your way, O Lord; lead me in a straight path . . . .*

PSALM 27:11 (NIV, 1984)

Questions

Have you ever prayed for your health?

☐ Yes ☐ No

If Yes, what have you prayed? If No, why not?

_____

_____

_____

DAY 3
Seeking Help

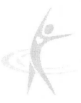

Scripture

³ *When you ask, you do not receive, because you ask with wrong motives, that you may spend what you get on your pleasures.*

JAMES 4:3 (TNIV)

Devotional

In January, the first month of the year, everyone wants to lose weight.

Perhaps it is because the doctor has mentioned that you need to lose weight, or maybe you are losing it for that cruise or to get into your wedding dress. Possibly it is because your family has noticed you have gained or because you think losing weight will get you that man.

We ask God to help us for the wrong reasons. We were made in his image, so why is everyone trying to change their image?

Yes, losing weight to become healthy or to stay healthy is a good thing. Losing weight to stay healthy and honor God's temple is even better.

First, seek God's help and set realistic goals. For example, losing five pounds a month is better and more realistic than trying to lose five pounds in one day.

Second, pray to God to send you an accountability partner. A partner can hold you responsible for cutting back on fat, decreasing your portion sizes, and making sure you exercise. Find a partner—a colleague, friend, or family member—you can trust and who lives by God's Word.

Prayer

Dear Heavenly Father, direct us on the paths that lead us to honor this temple you gave us. And, dear Father, give us instruction and direction to depend on one another according to your Word.

Brown-Bag Lunches— God Will Provide

Scripture

⁹ *For He satisfies the longing soul, And fills the hungry soul with goodness.*

PSALM 107:9 (NKJV)

Devotional

Putting God first will make you strive for his guidance and direction. This happened to me when I first declared Jesus as my savior. I wanted to read every book I could find about Jesus. I went to church every Sunday and to every meeting. My soul thirsted for knowledge, but I had to be sure I got the right knowledge and information.

This is true, too, for young adults when they become parents. They want their children to have the right food and beverages so they can be healthy and strong. During the months of August and September, millions of parents are contemplating what to fix their children and themselves for lunch. Is it peanut butter again?

Do not panic. I'm going to give you seven tips on how to add some pizzazz to your brown-bag lunches.

Prayer

Dear Heavenly Father, thanks for "The First Brown-Bag Lunch" when you fed over five thousand on five loaves of bread and two fish, and you gave them spiritual food, too. So, whenever I say grace over my food, I think of being blessed both spiritually and physically.

Activity

Brown-Bag Tips

TIP # 1

For condiments, use mustard and low-fat dressings such as nonfat yogurt mixed with your child's special seasonings.

Mix tofu with low-fat yogurt and add herbs to give the condiment flavor. You can also add salsa or vinegars.

If your children really love mayonnaise, then try low-fat or the eggless version.

TIP # 2

Add cut or sliced vegetables and/or apple wedges. Apple wedges may turn brown after slicing. You can sprinkle them with lemon juice or orange juice to prevent browning.

Alongside the vegetable or apple slices, include low-fat string cheese and low-fat pudding.

TIP # 3

To add taste and texture, try coleslaw mixed with pineapple and/or diced apples. You will not miss the fat from the mayonnaise.

TIP # 4

Do you have to have bread with your sandwiches? Roll up chicken salad or tuna fish salad in a romaine lettuce leaf. This is a great way to consume more vegetables.

TIP # 5

Roll thin slices of low-fat turkey or chicken around carrot or celery sticks. You can dip them in your favorite low-fat sauce.

TIP # 6

Make your own hummus and serve with warm pita bread. Two tablespoons of hummus equals 140 calories.

Stir-fry vegetables in olive oil and place them inside whole wheat pita bread.

You can buy seasoned olive oils. Try http://www.saporeoilandvinegar.com/index.html. I love their Italian blend.

The Brown-Bag Lunch Mix

For protein sources, try

- peanut butter
- low-fat turkey or chicken luncheon slices
- low-fat cheeses
- beans or tofu
- hummus

For breads, try

- whole wheat bagels
- whole wheat pita
- rye
- pumpernickel
- For an extra-light lunch on the go, try
- celery sticks with low-fat cream cheese and raisins (or craisins) on top; you can also sprinkle on granola
- a tomato stuffed with tuna or chicken salad
- tuna fish with five whole wheat crackers

- Lean Cuisine™ lunches; they are great, ranging from 220 to 500 calories and low in fat; however, the sodium is moderate to high, so look for meals with less than 550 mg. of sodium
- carrot sticks or a one-ounce serving of trail mix, for a snack packed in your lunch

Accountability Partner

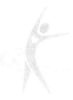

Scripture

[9] *Two are better than one, because they have a good return for their labor:* [10] *If they fall down, they can help each other up. But pity those who fall and have no one to help them up!*

ECCLESIASTES 4:9-10 (TNIV)

Devotional

Do you remember when you first joined church, they assigned you a prayer/spiritual partner? That person was someone you could call on when you needed help in reading the Bible or outside of church. That person was always there for you.

Find a similar partner you can trust and who can help guide you in the right directions toward living a healthy life with God's Word as your marker.

Our God is by our side each and every day; we may not see nor feel him, but God is there leading us on a right path. All you have to do is ask God and he will take you by the hand.

Prayer

Dear Heavenly Father, I can no longer walk this journey myself; I cry out for help. Please take my hand, so I will not be afraid to walk.

Questions

It is funny how we buy pills, powders, liquids, or even just starve ourselves to lose weight, but we are afraid to ask professionals for help.

Were you successful when you tried to change your eating habits by yourself?

☐ Yes ☐ No

If Yes, how long were you able to walk that journey? If No, why not?

_____

_____

_____

Did you go to TOPS™, Weight Watchers™, etc.?

☐ Yes ☐ No

If Yes, how long did you stick to your diet plan?

_____

_____

_____

Why did you stop?

_____

_____

_____

Pray on breaking down that pattern.

DAY 6
Getting Ready

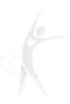

Scripture

⁴⁰ But all things should be done with regard to decency and propriety and in an orderly fashion.

1 Corinthians 14:40 (AMP)

Devotional

In order to eliminate some stress in your life, consider having a plan with action steps that will help you get to your destination. Plan with three goals in mind and set a deadline and boundaries. Keep God in your plans and pray that things will be according to his Word.

Why? You will be a better servant and be more disciplined in carrying out God's work.

Planning according to God's Word will give you

- less unnecessary stress
- more energy to do other things
- help in valuing yourself

- help in having others value and respect you

Prayer

Dear Heavenly Father, I pray for peace. Why? Because it will help me organize my life in all areas.

Activity

Why is order important for this journey?
- Keeping a food and exercise journal will help you stay on the course.
- You will be more alert.
- Your journey will not be as long when things are done in an orderly way.
- You will identify the causes that lead you to overeating.
- Having your steps in order will help propel you into the next journey of your life.

Record your food and exercise daily. Here's a sample diary to get you started.

Food & Exercise Diary

Mon	Tues	Wed	Thurs	Fri	Sat	Sun
Breakfast	Breakfast	Breakfast	Breakfast	Breakfast	Breakfast	Breakfast
Lunch	Lunch	Lunch	Lunch	Lunch	Lunch	Lunch
Snack	Snack	Snack	Snack	Snack	Snack	Snack
Dinner	Dinner	Dinner	Dinner	Dinner	Dinner	Dinner
Exercise	Exercise	Exercise	Exercise	Exercise	Exercise	Exercise

DAY 7

Cutting Back on Fat

Scripture

³⁴ *Therefore do not worry about tomorrow, for tomorrow will worry about itself. Each day has enough trouble of its own.*

MATTHEW 6:34 (NIV)

Devotional

Most of us hang on to the "worry" a lot. We worry about money and relationships. We worry if we will still have our jobs tomorrow and if we have enough food to feed our children.

But worrying doesn't add a minute, an hour, or a day to our lives, so why do we worry? If we have a problem, then let God handle it. There is no problem too big for God. Yet, we continue to worry until we realize nothing has changed. Then we cry out for Jesus's help. As a matter of fact, we should pray before every decision we make. Pray continuously without stopping. God hears our prayers, so pray and ask for his help. **Stop directing God and let God direct you.**

Ten years ago, there was a WAR on fat. Studies had shown fat in our diet can contribute to heart disease and some cancers. So the medical society, full steam ahead, formed a campaign to tell people to cut back on fat. Soon, the food industry followed. Now there are more low-fat products on the market than ever.

However, it is better to learn how to cut back fat for yourself than to rely on these low-fat products. God gave you the ability to choose. Let's learn how to choose low-fat products and make the right choice and stop worrying about it.

Prayer

Dear Heavenly Father, thanks for supplying all my needs.

Activity

Fat is an essential nutrient our body needs; it supplies us with energy. Fat also helps regulate body temperature and flavors food. Every gram of fat equals nine calories.

For example:

½ cup of ice cream

=

5 grams of fat

=

45 calories.

(9 calories x 5 grams of fat = 45 calories)

Ten Ways to Cut Back

1. Eat only six-ounce servings of lean meat, poultry, seafood, and cheese.

2. Use Benecol™, Smart Balance™, or Take Control™ instead of butter.

3. Eat more plant foods, vegetables, legumes, peas, and beans.

4. Eat more whole wheat cereals and pastas.

5. Bake, broil, stir-fry. Use vegetable sprays.

6. Read food labels.

7. Split high-fat entrées.

8. Order dressings, sauces, and gravies on the side.

9. Choose the low-fat versions of mayonnaise, salad dressings, and cheese.

10. When you use low-fat salad dressings, stick to the serving size.

Lower the calories but sizzle the senses by
- mixing collards with kale or mustard greens;
- adding tomatoes to black-eyed peas;
- adding low-sodium chicken broth to grits;
- making a low-fat yogurt cucumber sauce for fish or chicken;
- adding raisins to salads and coleslaw; and
- adding toasted nuts and raisins to rice to give it texture and crunchy taste.

DAY 8

Carbohydrates—
Good and Bad

Scripture

[12] *Apply your mind to instruction and correction and your ears to words of knowledge.*

Proverbs 23:12 (AMP)

Devotional

So many of my clients come to me after their fad diets have failed them. They have tried everything from the cookie to cabbage and pill diets. Yes, they work for a short time but offer no nutrient value. There is no substance in these diets.

After everything fails, *then* they look for someone who can give them instructions and the knowledge and the application to change their lifestyle. Funny, we do the same thing with God. Through his words we find instructions to live right and honor our temples, but we choose to do what we want until the bottom falls out. Only then do we

Carbohydrates—Good and Bad | 27

look for the expert or the instructions, and, most of all, only then do we call on God.

Below is some instruction on carbohydrates, which provide us with energy (glucose). Yet there are diets that restrict carbohydrates. Restriction leads to boredom and lack of nutrients and can lead to being moody. The next time you diet, limit your carbohydrates but do not restrict them so they are too low.

What Are Carbohydrates?

A **carbohydrate** is a nutrient that supplies us with energy. Every gram of carbohydrates equals four calories. They can be found in many different forms such as fruits, vegetables, whole grains, in some dairy products, and in some beverages.

There are two kinds of carbohydrates:

- **simple carbohydrates**—fruits, milk, jellies, jams, candies, cookies, and sweets

- **complex carbohydrates**—starches, fiber, and the skins of plants

Carbohydrates are important because they provide energy. The fiber part helps with the digestive tract. Carbohydrates are low in fiber and sugar and are a good source of vitamins, minerals, antioxidants, and phytochemicals which promote good health. The good carbohydrates can be found in whole wheat, grains, cereals, and rye bread, and in the skin of fruits.

However, white flour carbohydrates can raise blood sugar levels which, for persons with diabetes, can be harmful. The white starches quickly raise your blood sugar levels and, if not treated, can lead to complications for persons with diabetes.

Starchy beans, legumes, peas, and beans are starchy vegetables which are considered carbohydrates. The portion size recommended for peas and beans is ⅓ cup. They are a good source of protein when combined with rice and other beans or peas, but, if you have diabetes, remember to limit your amount.

How Much Should You Eat?
There is no recommended daily value; however, you do need anywhere from 50 to 100 grams per day (100 grams of carbohydrates = ⅓ cup).

Here are examples of the amount of carbohydrates in some common foods:

- one slice of bread = 15 grams
- ½ cup of orange juice = 15 grams
- ½ cup of rice = 15 grams
- ⅓ cups of beans = 15 grams

The National Academy of Science recommends 130 grams of carbohydrates per day to keep our brain cells alert.

Prayer

Dear Heavenly Father, I pray for wisdom so I can know what and how to eat, and how best to take care of my body.

Activity

Putting It All Together

Our meals should be balanced between proteins (meats, chicken, and fish) and carbohydrates (breads, cereals, pastas, fruit, and vegetables) and fats. Then add to this meal a low-fat dairy product and a low-fat, low-sugar dessert.

How do we lose weight? By eating fewer calories and increasing our exercise.

One pound of fat is equal to 3,500 calories, and, if we subtract 500 calories a day from our meal plan for seven days, that will be one pound (3,500) less of calories.

Getting Started

- Always eat a breakfast. The word *breakfast* means "break the fast." Since the night before you didn't eat anything while sleeping, start your day with energy. Rev up with a good meal.

- Choose more fresh foods and fewer processed foods because you will have better control over your portion sizes and ingredients.
- Drink plenty of water and fewer sodas. One can of regular soda can equal 150 calories. Imagine drinking four cans a day of soda, and you will be surprised how many calories you drink. Four sodas at 150 calories each equals 600 calories, and that is equal to one low-calorie meal.
- Eat three meals and a snack each day.
- Don't skip a meal, or you will overeat at the next meal.
- Be consistent and eat right for at least thirty days to help you develop a good habit.

DAY 9
Stop
Worrying

Scripture

²⁵ *"Therefore I tell you, do not worry about your life, what you will eat or drink; or about your body, what you will wear. Is not life more important than food, and the body more important than clothes?"*

MATTHEW 6:25 (TNIV)

Devotional

Sometimes, I feel people worry too much about their weight, especially if they do not have an illness related to their weight. The media have controlled our minds into thinking thin is IN. As a matter of fact, IN can be out because thin doesn't mean you are healthy.

God has given you a temple to take care of and to help serve others. Yes, he wants you to be healthy and strong, but not to the point where your body becomes your god and you place it before God in a manner that is not pleasing to him.

Worrying causes stress and stress makes us eat even more. If you cannot both eat right and exercise, then focus on one thing at a time.

Start the program you know you can accomplish and stick to it.

Prayer and reading God's Word will help you love yourself first. Start with the inside and it will take care of the outside.

Prayer

Dear Heavenly Father, help me to focus on you and not the things I cannot change.

Questions

What is holding you back from eating right?

Write down the actions you will take to knock down the obstacles/shackles keeping you from eating right.

Activity for the Next Seven Days

Walk by Faith

Walking is good for you. It is inexpensive and almost anyone can walk, though you should be sure to consult your doctor first. Once given the green light, go out for a walk. Test-walk first. Most people try to do three to five miles in one day, but that's too much to begin with, especially if you haven't exercised in years.

Work up to walking 10,000 steps a day; that will equal three miles. And when you achieve that, then slowly add additional steps.

Set a goal.

Grab a friend to walk with you.

Walk at the mall, but don't shop. Some malls have walking programs and give incentives for every twenty to fifty miles you complete.

Get a pedometer to help you keep track of miles or steps.

Winter Months

1. Be careful in the winter.

2. Dress warmly and in layers.

3. Because winter months can be cloudy, wear reflective clothing so drivers can see you.

4. Walk at the local school track.

Summer Months

1. Walk in the early evening or late afternoon, when it is cooler.

2. Wear appropriate clothes made of cotton because, when it becomes wet, it will hold the water and you can keep cool.

3. Wear the right shoes and change them every six months.

4. When your shoes become wet from the rain, let them dry with newspaper in them so they will dry faster and keep their shape.

5. Keep cool by carrying water with you.

6. If you have diabetes, always carry candy or Life Savers™ with you in case your blood sugar drops.

7. Be careful of listening to music because you may not hear the traffic.

8. Be aware of your surroundings.

And, in every season, most of all let someone know when and where you are going.

Start a walking program at church.

Reward the winners, not with food, but with movie tickets, a good book, or a gift card from a sports store.

Verses to Help You Meditate when You Walk

⁷ For we walk by faith, not by sight.

2 CORINTHIANS 5:7 (NKJV)

³ He told them: "Take nothing for the journey—no staff, no bag, no bread, no money, no extra shirt.

LUKE 9: 3 (TNIV)

⁹ In his heart a man plans his course, but the Lord determines his steps.

PROVERBS 16:9 (NIV1984)

¹⁴ I press toward the goal for the prize of the upward call of God in Christ Jesus.

PHILIPPIANS 3:14 (NKJV)

Walking Chart

On the next two pages is a Walking Chart. Keep track by miles, steps, or minutes. As long as you are consistent in your walking, you will see results in pounds dropping, inches falling off, or just feeling and sleeping better.

Get UP and Walk.

	Miles	Minutes	Steps
Monday			
Tuesday			
Wednesday			
Thursday			
Friday			
Saturday			
Sunday			

	Miles	Minutes	Steps
Monday			
Tuesday			
Wednesday			
Thursday			
Friday			
Saturday			
Sunday			

	Miles	Minutes	Steps
Monday			
Tuesday			
Wednesday			
Thursday			
Friday			
Saturday			
Sunday			

	Miles	Minutes	Steps
Monday			
Tuesday			
Wednesday			
Thursday			
Friday			
Saturday			
Sunday			

DAY 10
When to Say You've Had Enough

Scripture

[37] *All you need to say is simply 'Yes' or 'No' . . . .*

MATTHEW 5:37A (TNIV)

Devotional

When I was eight years of age, I used to asked for seconds and then third helpings of dinner. No one complained. My uncles and aunts would frown upon anyone who didn't ask for seconds. As a matter of fact, if you didn't ask for more, you didn't get invited back.

As I look back, it was okay to eat seconds and thirds because, afterward, we would go outside and play until the street lights came on. We also did household chores, including washing clothes by hand, dusting, changing linen, and washing floors. The whole family also participated in kickball, badminton, volleyball, and other physical activities.

Now these games are replaced with video games, which require you to sit in front of a screen. These and other changes have contributed to the obesity in American today, because one of the many factors leading to being overweight or obese is a sedentary lifestyle.

So let's begin by learning to say NO to video games on screen, on your phone, and at work. Let's go back to basics. Let's take walks after dinner and have a family membership at the gym instead of at the video shop.

Prayer

Dear Heavenly Father, help me to change my eating and exercise habits.

Questions

Take a look at your portion sizes. Are they huge?

☐ Yes ☐ No

Can you reduce the sizes?

☐ Yes ☐ No

If not, why not?

_____

_____

Here are some ways you can reduce your portions:

1. Cut them in half.

2. Reduce meat portion size to three ounces.

3. Have no more than 140 calories of a sweetened drink per week.

4. Eat no more than ten grapes.

5. Drink no more than ⅓ cup of dark juices (for example, blueberry, grape, and cranberry).

6. Eat no more than three whole eggs a week.

7. One-half of your plate should be fruits and vegetables.

8. One-fourth of your plate should be protein.

Can you think of anything else you can reduce?

_____

_____

_____

Portion Control

1 ounce of meat =
>   the size of a deck of cards

a medium apple =
>   about the size of a tennis ball

3 ounces of cheese =
>   a stack of four dice

½ cup of ice cream =
>   the size of a tennis ball

1 cup mashed potatoes =
>   about the size of a fist

1 teaspoon of butter, margarine, or peanut butter =
>   the size of the tip of the thumb

1 ounce of nuts =
>   one handful

Potato

1 small (3 oz.) =
>   80 Calories = 3 inches long or about ½ cup

1 medium (6 oz.) =
>   160 calories = 5 inches long

1 large (8 oz.) =
>   200 calories = 6 inches long

Fats

1 teaspoon margarine/butter =
    45 calories   = 1 pat

1 tablespoon mayonnaise =
    100 calories

2 tablespoons salad dressing =
    160 calories   = 1 small ladle (restaurant style)

DAY 11
If You Fail to
Make a Plan

Scripture

*⁹ In their hearts human beings plan their course, but
the Lord establishes their steps.*

PROVERBS 16:9 (TNIV)

Devotional

*If you fail to make a plan, then plan to fail. But you
cannot fail, when God is the pilot.*

Most of my friends have a visionary board. The
board is supposed to represent what they want in
life and the steps, in pictures, necessary to get to
their destinations. The idea is that, if you see your
vision every day, you will see your future.

Young girls see a wedding day in their dreams
and start planning before they have met their
princes. Young men who want to become bas-
ketball or football players start practicing and

visualizing their dreams every day. Entrepreneurs dream of making it big.

However, those dreams we see and plan for—are they on God's list? Do we plan with God or plan by ourselves?

Yes, we can dream and dream big, but who is laying down the course? When we don't get what we want, is it because of inadequate plans or because God has other plans for us?

I say: plan, pray, and put into action the steps God wants you to take. This applies to changing to a healthier lifestyle. Pray, plan with a purpose . . . and let God be your guide.

Prayer

Dear Heavenly Father, I pray to see the plan you have for me, and, even if I cannot see it, I pray to follow your will.

Questions

Have you ever jumped into a situation or an event or a project, only to find you have gotten in over your head?

☐ Yes   ☐ No

Did you then pray for God to get you out of the problem?

    ☐ Yes   ☐ No

Did you make a plan?

    ☐ Yes   ☐ No

If so, why did you not stick to your plan?

_____

_____

_____

Dining Out

The average American spends most of his food dollars outside the home. Buying breakfast, lunch, and dinner can cost your wallet plenty.

Just think: an average doctor's co-pay is $40, and you can spend close to that amount buying all three meals outside the home. An average breakfast meal is $6 plus tax. Then you buy a soda and a sandwich for lunch at $9 (depending upon where you live) and dinner, too, at an average of $20.

Wow! You just spend $35 dollars on fat, salt, and sugar. Doing this over a period of time can lead to obesity and the chronic illnesses that come with obesity.

It is possible to eat out and still make healthy choices?

Yes, and here are a few suggestions to get you started:

- Look at the fast-food or other restaurant's menu online and check the calories of their foods.
- Call ahead and see if the restaurant has a dieter's menu.
- Share an appetizer with a friend.
- Drink plenty of water to fill you before eating.
- Order salad with the dressing on the side.
- Share the high-fat entrée.
- Order a broth soup.
- Ask for sauces and gravies to be served on the side.
- Choose grilled, baked, broiled, boiled, or poached meats.
- Order steamed vegetables with sauces on the side.
- You now can download several diet calculator applications to your phone. Scan the food and it will tell you how many calories you are eating.

The Don'ts of Dining Out

- Don't go to a buffet, because they are loaded with calories, fat, salt, and sugar, and the temptation to overeat is great.
- Avoid the bread before the meal. It just provides extra calories.
- Always ask how the food is prepared.
- Avoid alcohol. Every ounce of alcohol is equal to seven calories. Why spend those extra calories on alcohol, when you can have an extra side of vegetables to fill you up?
- Share dessert or save it for later.
- If you order too much, ask for the to-go container and place half your food in the container or bag right away as a way of avoiding overeating.

DAY 12

Mastering Your Giants

Scripture

¹² *Everything is permissible (allowable and lawful) for me; but not all things are helpful (good for me to do, expedient and profitable when considered with other things). Everything is lawful for me, but I will not become the slave of anything or be brought under its power.*

1 CORINTHIANS 6:12 (AMP)

Devotional

We can go for ten days without water before our bodies start to deteriorate; however, we can go thirty days without food. I am not saying we should go without food and water. Our physical bodies need them in order to survive, but our spiritual bodies need living water, God's Word. We need both.

Food has become some people's addiction. Saying no to seconds and thirds is unheard of, and indulgence in other foods can lead us down the wrong path. This is not good for our temple.

Too much food can lead to unwanted calories, and, thus, we become overweight/obese. And our temples break down. Let Go and God.

Prayer

Dear Heavenly Father, help me knock down the giants that plague my mind and body.

Activity

For the next twenty-one days, throw away the salt shaker, caffeinated coffee, candies, cakes, cookies, and pies.

You will be surprised how much better you feel.

Replace

salt	with	herbs and spices
caffeinated coffee	with	decaffeinated coffee
candies	with	sugar-free Popsicles™
cakes, cookies, pies	with	fat- & sugar-free cakes, cookies, pies

If you have a sweet tooth, try unsweetened applesauce, sugar-free ice cream, or sherbet.

Water is an essential nutrient our body needs. Our bodies contain 50 to 70 per cent water. Our systems depend on water to function, and water keeps our body temperature cool.

Functions of Water

- flushes out toxins
- carries nutrients to our cells
- controls our body temperature
- acts as a cushion for some joints
- aids in digestion and elimination
- provides moistness for our nose, ears, and throat

How much do we need?

Men   —   6 to 13 cups a day
Women   —   4 to 9 cups a day

Or divide your body weight by two; that equals the number of ounces you need to drink in a day. For example, a 150-lb. person needs about 75 ounces, or approximately 9 cups (8 oz. = 1 cup).

When you deprive your body of adequate water, the following can occur:

- excessive thirst
- fatigue
- headache
- muscle weakness
- dehydration

If you exercise on a daily basis, you need to increase your water intake to replenish the amount lost while exercising. Drink four to six ounces before, during, and after exercise.

In hot climates, drink more to prevent heat exhaustion and to cool your body.

Illness or health conditions—such as fever, vomiting, or diarrhea—may require you to drink more water. Certain medications require you to drink more to prevent dryness in your mouth.

To get more water in your diet, eat more fruit and vegetables, such as watermelon, cucumbers, grapes, lettuce, and celery. Most people think if they drink more coffee, tea, or sodas, they are getting water in their diet. That's true; however, it is better to drink water alone without the added sugars or caffeine.

To get started, drink two glasses upon rising in the morning, two glasses at lunch, and two glasses at dinner.

DAY 13
Addictions

Scripture

⁵ *It is for freedom that Christ has set us free. Stand firm, then, and do not let yourselves be burdened again by a yoke of slavery.*

GALATIANS 5:1 (TNIV)

Devotional

Babies eat only when they are hungry, usually every four hours. Children eat when they are hungry, and, at times, may skip a meal or two. But, over the years, we learn to eat even when we are not hungry.

First, identify if you are eating because you are hungry, or because of your mood.

Some of us eat when we are lonely, sad, mad, depressed, and when we are happy.

The foods we eat at these times become what we call comfort foods.

Our emotions push us to eat, and, when we are satisfied, we become more calm and relaxed.

Research has shown that when the serotonin in our brain falls to a certain level, we tend to eat these foods. When it returns to normal, our brain sends a signal for us to become relaxed.

Some comfort foods are

- macaroni and cheese
- ice cream
- cake
- cookies
- brownies
- potato chips (salty and crunchy)

Yes, we need food to live, but some of us have taken food to a different level. Food has become our friend, and, at times, we are chained to food. It is our stronghold. You cannot release yourself from this stronghold; you need God to fix it. When food is an addiction, you alone cannot win.

Through prayer, meditation, and intervention, you can win. Call on God and your accountable partner to pull you through the storm.

This addiction hinders us from hearing, obeying, and loving God.

Prayer

Dear Heavenly Father, hear my cries and release this shackle that is binding me.

Questions

Are there some foods you have to eat?

_____

_____

Are there some foods you feel you cannot live without?

_____

_____

Can you replace them with nutrient-dense, low-calorie foods? Can you replace them with fruit, vegetables, unsweetened applesauce, water, or Crystal Light™?

☐ Yes ☐ No

Examine yourself. Look at your comfort food and replace it with a fruit and reading the Word. After a week, write down how you feel.

Replace the unhealthy with healthy choices. Instead of

ice cream	choose	yogurt
brownie	choose	one or two Hershey Kisses™ (lower in calories, but you can still have chocolate)
candy	choose	sugar-free, or Popsicles™

When depressed or mad, call a friend to vent. Call on your accountability partner.

And call on God to help you get through the storms of emotions.

DAY 14
Patience

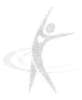

Scripture

[11] . . . *being strengthened with all power according to his glorious might so that you may have great endurance and patience, . . .*

COLOSSIANS 1:11 (TNIV)

Devotional

We all have heard the story about the tortoise and the hare (rabbit), a race between fast and slow. Isn't it funny that life is the same way?

We also see other people get the promotions, but soon they leave the job or something happens to make them leave the position. Or perhaps your friends get the big houses and big cars and you wish you had them, too. Perhaps you find yourself crying over the things you wish you had.

What does this have to do with the tortoise and the hare? The hare was very fast and sure of himself. He judged the tortoise by his size and his slow walk and talk. In fact, the hare took a nap. He let his guard down because he knew he was the fastest.

But we know who won the race—the tortoise—slow, but calculating and sure of himself. He took his time and got the prize. I want you to be patient on this journey. There is a saying, "Do it fast and it will not last." Do not rush through your journey or you will miss some steps and lose the prize.

Stay focused, call your accountability partner, and call on God.

Wait on some things before going to the next step. Revisit your goals.

Prayer

Dear Heavenly Father, I always rush through things, and, before you know it, they fall apart. I pray for patience and guidance and direction. Keep me on the path.

Activity

Turn off your phone, music, TV, and the radio. Next, light a candle and turn off the lights. Sit quietly and stare at the flame. Repeat these words:

"Peace; be still." Try to think of nothing but the flame.

Stare into the flame.

Notice how it flickers.

Take a deep breath.

Say, "Peace; be still."

Notice how the flame rises and falls.

It is the same with your journey, with its hills and valleys.

There is no straight road in life, but, with God's help, he will put you on the right path.

"Peace; be still."

Be patient; don't let your mind wander.

Take a deep breath.

"Peace; be still."

Have patience. With patience, you can endure the journey.

Look at the center of the flame. It is your inner strength . . . burning, flickering, blossoming. Don't put it out too soon.

Be patient.

Be strong.

Be resilient like the flame.

DAY 15

Working Smart

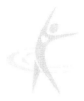

Scripture

[17] *Every part of Scripture is God-breathed and useful one way or another—showing us truth, exposing our rebellion, correcting our mistakes, training us to live God's way. Through the Word we are put together and shaped up for the tasks God has for us.*

2 TIMOTHY 3:17 (MSG)

Devotional

When we acknowledge that we need to change our eating and exercise habits, an action occurs. This is considered in the physical world, the pre-contemplation phase. In this phase, you admit you need to change and are searching for steps to reach the goal.

Some of us look for books, videos, audio materials, and classes to help with the process. Yet, for some of us, despite that, the connection is lost. Reading books to help you change your eating habits is great, but, if there is not action, the book is dead. There must be a mind-body-spirit connection to move you forward. The mind cannot hold the old habits and the good habits in the same space. Change occurs when you are willing to give up something. Are you willing to change to a healthier and more spiritual person?

Living by God's Word will shape and mold us to be better persons who will honor the temple he has given us. If you fall astray and become rebellious, read the Word. If you make mistakes, God will forgive you. Look for instruction; train by prayer, meditation, and listening to elders—all will keep you on the path.

Work smart by reading God's Word.

Prayer

Dear Heavenly Father, I pray not only that I see the words, but that I apply the words as well.

Questions

Have you ever bought books to help you diet?

☐ Yes ☐ No

Are you still using those books?

☐ Yes ☐ No

If not, why not?

_____

_____

_____

Buying and trying to get all the information on dieting can be confusing. Most all the books tell you something different, and I know that, for some people, they do not know where to begin. Seek God's direction and guidance, and look for a registered dietitian and personal trainer.

Activity for the Next Seven Days

Do fifty push-ups per day each Monday, Wednesday, and Thursday.

And don't forget to get in your 10,000 steps, too. As you begin each new activity, also continue with the previous week's activity.

DAY 16
The Wilderness

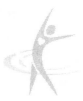

Scripture

37 For by your words you will be justified and acquitted, and by your words you will be condemned and sentenced.

MATTHEW 12:37 (AMP)

Devotional

We cannot be like the Israelites who traveled through the wilderness for forty years on a trip which should have taken nine days. Why did this happen? They traveled in circles because they didn't accept God's way. They wanted to get there in a hurry and they were looking for gold and riches. Does this sound familiar in your life?

Did you pray on it first? Or was your way the only way to get there and God was definitely not in your plans—until you needed him to get you out of a jam?

Perhaps you choose to use negative words: "I cannot exercise . . . I cannot diet . . . this is too hard." These words and choosing to do things your way will get you into trouble. God didn't plan for your journey to be peaceful and free of stress. He knew you would run into problems, but he is always by your side to help direct you and lead you down the path. The wilderness is not what God has in mind for you.

He created you in his image. He makes no mistakes. Yes, he gave us the ability to make a CHOICE; yet he wants you to rely on him, not your own will.

We cannot move from the wilderness when we hold on to old habits. Release and let go.

The next time you are given a choice, pray and ask for God's will, not yours. Get out of the wilderness.

Prayer

Dear Heavenly Father, I will always come to you first before I do things because, when I take things in my own hands, I circle in the wilderness trying to get out.

Questions

Our addiction to food is similar to being in the wilderness.

Addictions occur when you want everything your way.

Addictions occur when you eat to be full because you like the feeling of fullness.

Food becomes your god. And even drinking becomes your god.

Don't use these to cover up your pain. Remove those shackles.

Our emotions can take us to the wilderness.

So can lack of faith.

Holding on to grudges can take you there, too.

Can you identify your wilderness?

☐ Yes ☐ No

What changes can you make?

Why do you think some people prefer staying in the wilderness?

_____

_____

_____

How to Get Out of the Wilderness

1. Make a plan

2. Pray on the plan.

3. Select a friend to hold you accountable.

4. Look for a professional nutritionist or personal trainer.

5. Join or form a support group to help you get out of the wilderness.

DAY 17
Giving Up Is
Not an Option

Scripture

⁹ *Let us not become weary in doing good, for at the proper time we will reap a harvest if we do not give up.*

GALATIANS 6:9 (NIV)

Devotional

Learning something new can be challenging. Spending time trying to do it right can be stressful and tiring and drain our energy. When you have tried several times and still haven't accomplished your goal, frustration sinks in and you give up, give in, and give out.

STOP. Try one more time. It is not the destination that counts, but the steps you took and what you learned along the way. We all feel frustrated when we cannot achieve our goals, but look at the journey.

Measure how far you have come and gained along the way.

Through the sweat, tears, and pain, you have achieved some ground. Look at what you have learned and, then, what you didn't learn.

Keeping a food, exercise, and even mood diary will help you jump the hurdles and obstacles in the way of changing your eating and exercise habits.

Prayer

Dear Heavenly Father, I work and work and work for my dream, but there are times I want to give up. But I give thanks to you; you keep pushing me.

Activity

Take a CAT scan of your mind.

"CAT" stands for Control your Actions and Thoughts.

Learn to wait patiently and reap the harvest. There is a old saying: "Do it fast and it will not last."

Six Incentives/Methods to Help
You Take Your Time

1. You will make fewer mistakes.

2. Take a step back and revisit your goals.

3. You want to build a firm, solid foundation.

4. Before you quit, think of what you have accomplished.

5. Reward yourself for your hard work.

6. Think about the steps and not the destination.

DAY 18
Pressing Toward Your Goal

Scripture

[24] *Do you not know that in a race all the runners run, but only one gets the prize? Run in such a way as to get the prize.*

1 Corinthians 9:24 (TNIV)

Devotional

In sports, the athlete has to train hard to get the prize. He or she doesn't allow any distractions from their goal. It requires discipline and endurance to stay in a race to the finish. Perhaps a co-worker, family member, or friend wants to compete against you to lose weight. Good. A little competition doesn't hurt, as long as you keep your eyes on God.

In God's race, everyone gains a prize whether you win or lose. In the physical world, there is only one winner. Does this mean the others didn't train as hard? Don't beat yourself up because you didn't lose five pounds; you may have lost one pound or two. Did you gain knowledge about eating right while you were competing? In the spiritual world, it is not about winning the prize; it is about gaining God's love and developing a relationship with HIM. It is a race for the imperishable crown.

Run! God, will reward you for staying on the course and staying in the race.

Prayer

Dear Heavenly Father, I am ready to run the race.

Questions

Press toward your goal with God as the director. Press forward to receive your crown.

Your crown can be losing a certain number of pounds.

Your crown can be lowering your blood pressure.

Your crown can be lowering your blood glucose level.

What is your crown?

_____

_____

_____

Read 1 Corinthians 9:24-25. According to Paul, what do we get when we race for God?

Barriers to Exercise

Barrier	Then . . .
location (the gym is too far away)	hire a personal trainer; start a walking group.
need a baby-sitter	some gyms have a baby center; if the children are young enough to be placed in a carriage, run behind the carriage.
hair (don't want to sweat your curls out)	wear a wig or let your hair go natural.
"I am afraid of getting muscles."	be glad you have muscles; they are needed in order to lift, walk, and move; strengthening your muscles burns more energy and makes you look leaner.
"I don't want to exercise alone."	enjoy developing friendships if you go to a gym.
"I am too big to go to a gym; all the other women or men are smaller than me."	find a gym set aside for the larger person; work out with programs on TV; join a group like TOPS™, where you can find help with other large people.

Drop the excuses.

Why Should You Exercise?

- to prevent obesity, which can lead to heart disease, hypertension, diabetes, and bone disease
- to look and feel great
- to build self-esteem
- to build bone
- to sleep better
- to become more flexible
- to have more energy
- to slow down the aging process
- to build brain cells
- to build self-confidence
- to lower blood pressure
- to lower blood glucose levels
- to lower blood cholesterol levels

Keep Your Eyes on the Prize

Scripture

¹³ *Brothers and sisters, I do not consider myself yet to have taken hold of it. But one thing I do: Forgetting what is behind and straining toward what is ahead,* ¹⁴ *I press on toward the goal to win the prize for which God has called me heavenward in Christ Jesus.*

PHILIPPIANS 3:13-14 (TNIV)

Devotional

Run, run, for the prize. Yes, winning the prize is great, but the emotional peace lasts for only a short time. Soon it will all be forgotten, and then you have to train again to keep the prize. In the spiritual world, we run for God's love and a relationship with him.

In the physical world, the athlete trains every day, sometimes for hours. He or she has to keep the body strong. The day consists of training and eating right and staying away from those things that will distract him or her from the prize.

In the spiritual world, the disciplined "athlete" trains by reading, praying, meditating, and by fellowship with others like himself or herself to help gain the prize. He or she should avoid the distractions that keep them from the course. Eating and exercise should be included to keep the body strong and fit, so she or he can better serve God.

Prayer

Dear Heavenly Father, I will stay focused on going forward and not looking back at my past. Yes, I know I can learn from my past, but holding on to it will keep me from moving forward.

Questions

Are you staying on the course?

☐ Yes   ☐ No

If No, why have you drifted off the course?

_____

_____

_____

Name three things that can get you to train physically and spiritually.

_____

_____

_____

DAY 20
Renewing Your Strength

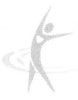

Scripture

[31] . . . *[B]ut those who hope in the Lord will renew their strength. They will soar on wings like eagles; they will run and not grow weary, they will walk and not be faint.*

ISAIAH 40:31 (TNIV)

Devotional

Putting old habits behind us can be hard. We all like the comfort of the familiar. Pressing forward into the unknown is scary. But let's face it: where you are right now was once the unknown, too— yet you made it through.

There may have been scratches, bruises, even pain, and we didn't know when or how, but we came through the storm. He will carry us through many challenges. "I will never leave you nor forsake you." (Hebrews 13:5, TKJV) God does things in an unnatural way. HE does things on his own time and not ours.

You have lost the weight, and now your friends notice you don't eat like you used to. They want to go out and eat after work, but are they afraid you will be bored?

Prayer

Heavenly Father, I will call on you every day for strength and courage.

Questions

Do you go out and eat the way you used to?

☐ Yes ☐ No

Or do you now go out and eat what is on your meal plan?

☐ Yes ☐ No

How would you handle this challenge?

_____

_____

_____

Go out and eat, but stick to your meal plan. If

your friends cannot accept your values, then they are not your friends.

How does God motivate you on this journey?

_____

_____

_____

Ways to Renew Your Mind

- Pray and work out with your spiritual partner.
- Take one day at a time.
- Set goals you can keep.
- Write, recite, and revisit your goals once a week.
- Keep a journal on your eating and exercising and also record your moods. This will be helpful because you will know what moods trigger you to overeat.
- Be positive and hang with positive people Winners will always bring out the best in you.

DAY 21
Step Back to Step Forward

Scripture

23 The Lord makes firm the steps of the one who delights in him; 24 though he may stumble, he will not fall, for the Lord upholds him with his hand.

PSALM 37:23-24 (NIV)

Devotional

We all have started a project, only to stop it a few days or weeks later because we failed to realize how much work we had to put into the project or how long it was going to take.

By now, you are probably wondering how many more days you have on this journey.

Questions are swimming in your head, including wondering if you really want to continue. But God didn't give up on you. If he had, where would you be? Although giving up is easy, God has plans for you. And I didn't say the journey would be easy. There are a lot of bad habits to destroy and shackles have to be burned.

God will not let you fall. As a matter of fact, there will be stumbling and missing a step or two, but God is there to catch and hold on to your hand.

This is the midpoint—time to reevaluate your progress. If you cannot exercise twenty minutes in a row every day, then change your action steps. Take ten minutes in the morning, ten minutes at lunch, and ten minutes after dinner. Believe it or not, you will still see the benefit when exercising for ten minutes at intervals throughout the day.

Don't give up or give in; you are halfway down the road.

Prayer

Dear Heavenly Father, I have fallen down so many times, but you were there to pick me up each time, and I am grateful. I pray that you will become my beacon of light so I will not stumble and fall because of distractions.

Questions

Have you every given up on your plan?

    ☐ Yes   ☐ No

If Yes, why?

_____

_____

If No, what makes you stay motivated?

_____

_____

How to Stay Motivated

To keep your mind from negative words and thoughts, try these few suggestions and ideas.

When You Think . . .	Instead, Think . . .
I want to eat the whole cake.	I will eat only a slice that is 1/8 of the cake.
I cannot exercise for an hour.	I will focus on one or two muscle groups for thirty minutes.
It is raining outside so I cannot go out and exercise.	I will put on a tape and walk indoors.
Here I am at the Christmas party and they have all the food I cannot eat. I will leave and go home early.	I am glad I brought my own food. I will focus on eating the fruit and vegetables and sip on seltzer water.
My walking partner is sick. I cannot go by myself.	I will walk indoors, in the hallways, or around the building, or at the mall (but I won't shop).
My coach will be mad at me, I only lost two pounds instead of five pounds.	Wow, I lost two pounds since last week.

Now write down the negative thoughts in your mind in the left column and change them to positive comments in the right column.

When You Think . . .	Instead, Think . . .

Not by Your Will but by HIS Will

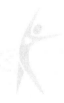

Scripture

⁹ *In their hearts humans plan their course, but the Lord establishes their steps.*

PROVERBS 16:9 (NIV)

Devotional

The day you were born, your parents had plans for you. They had established a formula for your life, and, if you obeyed and stayed on their course, you would not fall from their grace.

Then you went to school, where they had plans for you, too. And when you became of age, you had your own plans.

However, God has plans for you, too. Before you were conceived, he developed a plan which included protection, guidance, direction, caring, and love, and, in turn, you became a soldier for God.

Our plan is to honor God, to respect and serve and practice the "fruits of the Spirit"— love, joy, peace, patience, kindness, goodness, faithfulness, gentleness, and self-control. (See Galatians 5:22-23.)

But, like children, we want to do things our way until we cannot fight any more. Come home.

Prayer

Dear Heavenly Father, I will obey and trust you because you know what is best for me.

Questions

How many days did you follow your healthy lifestyle plan?

Why didn't you follow your plan the other days?

What happened when you didn't follow your plan?

Activity For The Next Seven Days

Do at least fifty sit-ups or crunches each Monday, Wednesday, and Thursday, and don't forget to continue the activities begun in previous weeks.

DAY 23
Let It
Go

Scripture

²¹ *Little children, keep yourselves from idols (false gods)—[from anything and everything that would occupy the place in your heart due to God, from any sort of substitute for Him that would take first place in your life]. Amen (so let it be).*

I JOHN 5:21 (AMP)

Devotional

Have you ever had a friend who tried to direct your life? Told you what to wear, how to eat, what to do, and how to speak?

It is good to have friends look after you, but your life is your life to live and not theirs to control. The same applies to you. We all want the best for each other, but we should not try to control each other.

God wants the best for us, too; yet he gave us the ability to choose. He wants us to follow HIS words and obey them, but he also knows we don't always choose his way.

And still, if you fall down, he is there to pick you up and send you on your way. He doesn't hold any grudges or keep account of our wrongs. He loves us no matter how many times we fall.

Sometimes our friends fail to pick us up. Be careful: not everyone has your health in mind. Wait on God for your answers and not on your friends.

All God wants is for us to focus on HIM and keep him in the decision-making process as we press forward to our goal.

Prayer

Dear Heavenly Father, I pray you will send me people who want me to follow you and not them.

Questions

Since this journey began, have you prayed on your walk?

☐ Yes ☐ No

If not, why not?

_____

_____

_____

Do you have an accountability partner?

☐ Yes ☐ No

Are you and your partner praying about the journey?

☐ Yes ☐ No

Studies have shown that, when people hold each other accountable for a goal, they are more likely to succeed. Don't be afraid to ask your doctor, nutritionist, or personal trainer. They can help you decide which way to travel toward your healthy lifestyle goal.

Activity

Reflect on your progress. Be aware of those fad diets that tell you to eliminate a lot of foods from your diet. They do work, but only for a short period of time. Take notes on how far you have come and what you have accomplished. Pat yourself on the back.

Don't blame yourself if you didn't lose the weight you wanted. Focus on what you have learned.

Don't throw in the towel until you have exhausted all avenues.

If you go back to your old habits for one day, re-member: you can get back up and start over again.

And, if you haven't met your goals, maybe your goals were not realistic. Revisit, rewrite, and recite your goals.

DAY 24
Do Not Fear

Scripture

¹³ *For I am the Lord your God who takes hold of your right hand and says to you, Do not fear; I will help you.*

ISAIAH 41:13 (TNIV)

Devotional

When you go through change, you will have to give up an old behavior and replace it with a good behavior. The reason most of us do not change is fear of the unknown. You may be afraid your friends will no longer like you, but, mostly, finding the real you can be scary.

Don't be afraid to cut back on fats and replace them with herbs and spices.

Don't be afraid to switch from whole milk to 1% milk; you will gain more muscle than fat.

Don't be afraid to replace whole eggs with egg whites.

Don't be afraid to cut back on calories—and add years to your life.

Don't be afraid to cut back on sweets and replace them with sugar-free products.

Don't be afraid to cut back on cookies; there are sugar-free cookies that taste twice as good but have fewer calories.

Prayer

Dear Heavenly Father, I entered the path without knowing what the end will bring; however, if you take my hand, I will not be afraid.

Fear stands for False Evidence Appearing Real

The next few days, I will focus on strength, power, faith, and *fear*.

The reason so many of us fail to continue on our journey is the fear of failure. You have been on so many diets and exercise programs, only to have quit after a few months.

Or perhaps you quit because an event or situation stopped you in your tracks. Don't be alarmed, but there are a lot of people who do not want you to succeed.

Be wary of distraction, focus on God, remember to train in the spiritual, and the physical world will fall in place. Giving up or giving in is not an option with God.

DAY 25
He Gives
Me Strength

Scripture

²⁹ *He gives strength to the weary and increases the power of the weak.*

ISAIAH 40:29 (NIV)

Devotional

In the first few days of dieting, one loses water and some inches. Everyone is excited and works even harder, but then all the hard work stops because, for one or more weeks, the weight doesn't change, the inches remain the same. Then it hits you: you have reached a plateau, and, the harder you work, the more you remain the same.

Then a lapse period begins. This is when you go back to your old habits. It is like a dance. You dance between the old habits and the new habits. The journey doesn't excite you anymore, and soon you find yourself staying more with the bad habits.

This is natural for a lot of people, but there are others who kick, scream, cry, and push through that plateau, onward to winning the prize.

Why? What is the difference between those who quit and those who keep going?

Perseverance . . . keeping focus yet remaining flexible . . . knowing the plateau is only temporary . . . revisiting goals . . . all of those help. But, most of all, the ones who keep going know their power to overcome obstacles is through God.

They are not stronger than the quitters. The winners simply know when they cannot fix it, so they call upon God. They will admit they are weak and cry out for God. They will fall down to their knees and pray, in the good and bad times.

Prayer

Dear Heavenly Father, my storm is hard and rough. Show me your hand.

Question

Do you have a scripture or song that will give you strength? Write it here and revisit it when you feel weak.

DAY 26
Fear or Faith

Scripture

[25] *To fear anyone will prove to be a snare, but whoever trusts in the Lord is kept safe.*

PROVERBS 29:25 (TNIV)

Devotional

Which do you choose?

Mr. Postman, send fear back; it doesn't live here anymore?

With change come hesitation, doubt, and fear.

But when God is in your corner, you come out fighting. Remember when you felt strong when your big brother or sister protected you from bullies? You felt as if you had all the POWER in the world with you.

Shake it, punch it, fight it—embrace your fear and overcome it.

If fear gets through, it is because you allowed it. With faith as your shield, nothing will harm you.

Prayer

Dear Heavenly father, please hold my hand as I tread new waters.

DAY 27
No Pain, No Gain

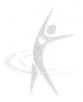

Scripture

³ . . . *[We] also glory in our sufferings, because we know that suffering produces perseverance . . .*

ROMAN 5:3 (TNIV)

Devotional

This scripture passage states that, through our many trials and tribulations, we develop patience. Life consists of many trials, and, the more we go through the storm of life, the more we develop endurance and patience.

There is no way or avenue to hurry the storms in our lives. First we must embrace them. Look at them as positive markers to help us on our journey. It is through the pain our passion blossoms.

Yes, even when you are dieting and exercising, there is some pain. And in the end we rejoice because we have accomplished our goals.

So, for this lesson, I want you to challenge your temple with increasing your exercise program.

If you are walking 10,000 steps, then move up to 15,000. Instead of 150 sit-ups, increase to 180.

Increase your push-ups to five sets of ten. Do a set in the morning, afternoon, evening, and before going to bed.

Prayer

Dear Heavenly Father, I have traveled down this road, I have felt the pain, and I have endured.

Activity

Increase your workout.

Do heavy work four days a week, and three days of cardio for an hour-and-a-half.

No more excuses.

Is Eight Hours of Sleep Enough?

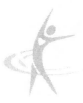

Scripture

[28] *"Come to me, all you who are weary and bur-dened, and I will give you rest. . . ."*

Matthew 11:28 (TNIV)

Devotional

Are you getting eight hours of sleep? Your body needs rest to help rejuvenate and renew the body's cells. Trying to burn the candle at both ends does not work. You'll find your brain cannot rejuvenate the cells needed to function. Your memory short-ens and the capability to do things decreases.

The less you sleep, the greater your chance of early mortality.

Studies have shown, if your body doesn't get rest, you can gain weight, develop high blood pressure, and become less mentally sharp, com-pared to when you get enough sleep.

Prayer

Dear Heavenly Father, I notice when I follow your plans, I have enough energy because I don't worry at night. I sleep well when I let you direct my path.

Activity

Sleep Stealers
- stress and depression
- caffeine
- smoking
- exercising too close to bedtime
- your partner's snoring
- unusual work hours
- going through menopause
- pain
- sleep apnea (a common disorder in which you have one or more pauses in breathing or take shallow breaths while you sleep)

What can you do? Set up a sleeping ritual.

First, your bedroom should be just that: a place where you sleep. If your bedroom serves as an office, too, definitely turn the fax off and take all business papers off the bed.

Here are some other tips:

- Shut off the television, radio, and phone.
- Take a long bath surrounded by candles.
- Drizzle essential oils in your bath water. (Lavender makes you sleepy; cardamom and wintergreen make you calm and relax your muscles.)
- Brush your teeth.
- Put on some warm pajamas.
- Go to bed the same time (if you can) every night.
- Avoid taking long naps during the day, or you may not be able to sleep at night.
- Don't go to bed if you are not sleepy.
- Make sure the temperature of the room is right for you.
- Turn off the lights; having lights on disturbs your natural sleep rhythms.
- Don't go to bed either hungry or having eaten a large meal right before.

This schedule will prepare you for a good night's sleep. If you do this ritual for the next twenty-one days, you will build a good habit.

Activity for the Next Seven Days

Buy a hula hoop. It is great for the waistline.

Instructions:

1. Place the hula hoop on the ground.
2. Step into the hula hoop.
3. Lift the hoop above your ankles to your waistline.
4. Hold the hoop against your back.
5. With both hands, swing the hoop toward the left side.
6. Move your hips in a circular motion.
7. When the hoop is moving in a circular motion, it should be touching your back and abdomen.
8. Keep your feet planted tight on the ground.
9. Your movement is through the hips and not the feet.

DAY 29
Finding the Hidden Treasures

Scripture

[13] *I can do all things through Christ who strengthens me.*

PHILIPPIANS 4:13 (NKJV)

Devotional

Deadlines . . . proposals, and a midterm to write . . . all by Friday . . . phew.

Whether it is on paper or in your head, whether it is taking care of your children or your parents, it can all be overwhelming. This is called stress.

Stress can be internal or external forces that raise your blood pressure and heart rate, and even make you sick if not treated. In fact, stress over a period of time can lead to anxiety attacks and even depression.

Most people think when you become a Christian, there is no longer stress in your life. Everything is now peaches and cream. But no. We all have stress; it is a way of life. How you look at it and handle it will determine if it is negative or positive.

However, when you read the Bible, meditate, and pray every day, you can prevent stress or at least keep your stress level down.

Lack of sleep can make you feel tired during the day and can contribute to your making wrong food choices. Call on God for strength. This does not mean you can still do one hundred things at the same time, but it does mean that, when you feel you cannot go on, you can call on God for strength.

Developing a relationship with God can help you see things differently and look for divine order in chaos.

Pray continuously.

Prayer

Dear Heavenly Father, I thank you for the strength you have given me. All the power I have comes from you.

Questions

Where do you get your power when things look bad?

_____

_____

_____

DAY 30
Refuge

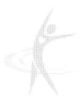

Scripture

8 O taste and see that the Lord [our God] is good! Blessed (happy, fortunate, to be envied) is the man who trusts and takes refuge in Him.

PSALM 34:8 (AMP)

Devotional

The dictionary says refuge means shelter or protection from danger or distress.

Take refuge in God, and release all things unto HIM. Carrying the extra baggage only slows you down and you will have to work twice as hard to get to your destination.

Leave the baggage at the altar.

Stress makes you overeat, drink to excess, and even spend too much money on such things as buying clothes and shoes or anything you do not need. These do not help you to grow emotionally, physically, and spiritually.

Put your trust in God, take refuge, and ask for help.

Prayer

Dear Heavenly Father, learning how to eat and exercise can be challenging, but I know you are there for me.

Activity

Write in your journal to help get stressful thoughts out of your mind

Write Your Stress Away

DAY 31
Stress to the Max

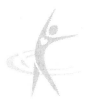

Scripture

²⁸ *You, Lord, keep my lamp burning; my God turns my darkness into light.*

PSALM 18:28 (TNIV)

Devotional

The holidays for some people are very painful because of having lost a loved one through death, divorce, or separation. And losing your job or home can be stressful on you and your family.

What or whom do reach for?

> *Why, my soul, are you downcast? . . .*
> *Put your hope in God . . .*
> — PSALM 42:11 (TNIV)

Stressful times test our faith. Why do some people smile through hard times and others give in and give up?

Perhaps it is FAITH, your relationship with God. Researchers have studied faith and medicine and found those who get through a terminal illness relied on faith. Your mind is a powerful weapon when it feels threatened. The body release endorphins to help you either fight or flee. Either you stay and fight, or you run.

Run toward your giants because God is with you. Let your faith become your shield and courage your sword. Meet the situation head on with a positive attitude that "this too shall pass," and you will win.

Know your ABCs:

A. be **A**ware; **A**cknowledge the situation or event

B. **B**elieve, even though you know you cannot change the situation or event you can change the way you look at the event

C. **C**ommit to change your attitude; change how you see things

And know you cannot change A, but you can change B—and B changes C.

Prayer

Dear Heavenly Father, I will continue to seek peace and see things through your eyes and not mine.

Questions

Can you identify the stressors in your life? Are you

- bored?
- separated from a love one?
- worried about bills?
- dealing with a lack of money?
- unhappy in your job?
- in a new location?

Can you think of others?

With prayer and meditation and conviction, you can get through the storm. Ride the waves and wind and hear Jesus say, "Peace; be still," and watch how the storms in your life become ripples on a pond.

Have you ever gone through a storm in your life and wondered how you were going to get out? After you did, did you then look back and wonder, "Did I really go through that storm?"

What did you do to help you get through the storm?

_____

_____

_____

Who helped you?

_____

_____

_____

DAY 32
Embrace the Struggle

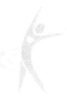

Scripture

²² *A cheerful heart is good medicine, but a crushed spirit dries up the bones.*

PROVERBS 17:22 (NIV)

Devotional

You've probably heard this story a hundred times, the one about two men sitting on a porch with an old slender dog? While the two men are talking, the dog keeps whining.

One man says, "What is wrong with your dog? Is he sick?"

The other man says, "He is lying on a nail. And all he has to do is move two inches to the left and he will stop whining."

Does this sound like someone you know? They are crying, whining, or complaining all the time, but all they have to do is move away from the situation or event or person and everything will be fine.

Does it sound like you?

People who are always cheerful tend to attract people who are cheerful, but the one who is always frowning, complaining, and whining—well, people tend to stay away from folks like that.

On your journey, some people will try to sabotage you by being negative or even by offering you foods not on your meal plan. Stay away from them because they will wear you down.

The same applies when you first start going to church. You will have people who will say negative things about you or try to tell you jokes that are not clean, just to see your response. Put them on your delete list.

Unclutter those unnecessary e-mails or phone calls and those things that do not belong on your to-do list. Hang around the champions, the winners, because they want you to have the best.

Prayer

For today's prayer, I am using Romans 8:26 from *The Message*, but I have placed "I/me/my" in the passage so you can read it, internally, as meant for you.

Dear Heavenly Father, meanwhile, the moment I get tired in the waiting, God's Spirit is right alongside helping me along. If I don't know how or what to pray, it doesn't matter. He does my praying in and for me, making prayer out of my wordless sighs, my aching groans. . . .

Activity

Things to Do to Stay Positive
- Repeat affirmations.
- Read your Bible.
- Go to church.
- Listen to gospel music.
- Do deep-breathing exercises.

DAY 33
Release the Past

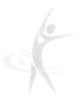

Scripture

[18] *"Forget the former things; do not dwell on the past."*

ISAIAH 43:18 (TNIV)

Devotional

There is nothing wrong with learning from the past; however, keep the past baggage in the past. Dancing back and forth is not healthy for your body, mind, or soul. It only reminds you of the hurts and pain.

Release those strongholds of bad habits. Get rid of negative things.

When you focus too much on the bad, your hurts and pains become your GOD, and your mind will not rest. Eventually your body can break down, and you can end up with colds, illnesses, and fatigue.

In Psalms, David says to God, renew my mind . . . give me a clean heart, mind, and soul.

Being afraid of the future is normal; we all have been there. Look at yourself TODAY; think of all the knowledge you have acquired, things you didn't know years ago or even last year. Trust in God. Have faith and let God lead you.

As my mother used to say, "This too shall pass."

Prayer

Dear Heavenly Father, thanks for the memories, but I am moving to a better place.

DAY 34
Purpose Driven

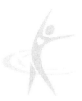

Scripture

[16] *So I say, walk by the Spirit, and you will not gratify the desires of the sinful nature.* –

GALATIANS 5:16 (TNIV)

Devotional

Wow! You are almost through the 40 days of your spiritual and physical journey. Coming this far means you are driven to change your lifestyle. You have given a purpose to starting new.

When you are purpose driven, nothing can stop you. There will be a couple of relapses, but you have all the tools needed to get back on the path and continue. The same is true of using this book; now you can go back and start anywhere and still be able to stay on the path.

Remember to rewrite your goals, then recite and revisit them . It is not the destination that counts: it is the steps along the way that will help you build the temple.

Prayer

Dear Heavenly Father, thanks for the power, love, and instruction because I can only move in your direction.

Activity

How Can You Keep Going?

- Continue to make a journal of your journey.
- Stay focused.
- Researchers say, when you teach someone and they in turn take the material and teach someone else, the information will stay with you. So, teach your family how to eat right!
- If you take the information and do it for thirty days, you will develop good habits. Don't break the chain.
- Make short-term goals. And call your goals *lifestyle goals*; that makes them easier to achieve.
- Have someone hold you accountable.
- Rewrite, recite, and revisit your lifestyle goals.

- And, most of all, know that a healthy lifestyle can build a healthy temple, and you *will* become a better servant in body, mind, and spirit.

DAY 35
Training Hard

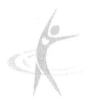

Scripture

[11] *No discipline seems pleasant at the time, but painful. Later on, however, it produces a harvest of righteousness and peace for those who have been trained by it.*

HEBREWS 12:11 (TNIV)

Devotional

Purpose driven people seek out their goals, train to achieve them, and then live them. They do not have a Plan B because they have already asked GOD for his help and his direction. So, they are physically and spiritually trained to have a strong, healthy body, mind, and spirit.

In the physical world, exercise three to five times a week for thirty minutes or longer. Bones and muscles are strengthened by lifting weights. Then train your heart and lungs with walking or running. And supplement all this with eating right.

In the spiritual world, train by reading and listening to the Word. Fellowship with other Christians. Praying everyday is not optional because it builds up faith and hope.

Both the physical and spiritual need discipline and direction to yield a good disciple.

Just as a car needs a tune-up every 15,000 miles, our spirits and physical bodies need a tune-up, too. The tune-up is getting rid of doubt, lack of faith, negativity. Every day, you must train hard to build the temple God has given you.

Prayer

Dear Heavenly Father, thanks for everything.

The Sovereign Lord is my strength;
he makes my feet like the feet of a deer,
he enables me to tread on the heights.
— HABAKKUK 3:19 (NIV)

Activity for the Next Seven Days

Get out the jump rope. Jump with family members or by yourself.

DAY 36
The Last
Supper

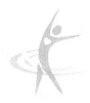

Scripture

⁵⁻⁹ So don't lose a minute in building on what you've been given, complementing your basic faith with good character, spiritual understanding, alert discipline, passionate patience, reverent wonder, warm friendliness, and generous love, each dimension fitting into and developing the others. With these qualities active and growing in your lives, no grass will grow under your feet, no day will pass without its reward as you mature in your experience of our Master Jesus. Without these qualities you can't see what's right before you, oblivious that your old sinful life has been wiped off the books.

2 PETER 1:5-9 (MSG)

Devotional

You can change your attitude, and, with the new attitude, a new behavior rises. All it takes is discipline to strengthen your faith, just as it takes training and discipline to train your body.

Moving from bad habits to good habits requires strength. Call on GOD; you cannot do it alone. Praying, meditating, reading, and fellowship with others help to mold and shape you into a soldier for God's army. All these are not for just a moment but for a lifetime, just as, for a lifetime, we are supposed to nurture, feed, and provide water to our bodies so they may grow and become strong.

But, for some unknown reason, we are reluctant to follow God's work and his plan for us. We want to hold on to our bad habits.

When I get a call from new clients, the first words from their mouths are, "This is my last supper; before I come to you, I am going to eat as much as I can."

I was thinking about *the* Last Supper, when Jesus spent time with his disciples, breaking bread and drinking wine. This is the night of his betrayal, the night before the denial of who he IS.

When I started writing this book, I wondered if you will say the same thing: "This is my last supper."

Do you think I will deny you eating your favorite foods?

I want you to think of *your* last supper not as about denying you foods, but giving you foods from the garden, foods that will enrich your mind, body, and spirit and prevent disease.

Is this your "last supper"?

- sugar
- fat
- salt
- fatty desserts
- huge portion sizes
- no exercise
- junk food
- dining out
- fast food
- TV
- stress
- alcohol
- Sodas
- Lack of Sleep
- Partying
- Depression

Your new "last supper" should look like this after 40 days:

- sugar-free
- fat-free
- low-salt
- fresh fruit for dessert (low in fat and sugar)
- smaller portion sizes
- water
- praying daily (living water)
- no junk food
- healthy dining out
- healthy fast foods
- limits on TV
- physical activity

- stress management techniques
- Drinking more water(helps you physically), but should thirst for the living water too.

These things equals a more healthier physical and spiritual YOU.

Prayer

Dear Heavenly Father, I am grateful for this temple you gave me and I will honor it.

DAY 37
New Attitude

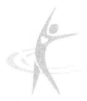

Scripture

[11] " . . . *For I know the plans I have for you,*" *declares the Lord,* "*plans to prosper you and not to harm you, plans to give you hope and a future.*"

JEREMIAH 29:11 (NIV)

Devotional

I have seen people change their attitudes and behaviors when they lose weight, as if something inside has emerged on the scene. They carry a different tune and the light around them shines. Their outlook on life changes and soon they find themselves floating.

These people are no longer carrying the excess baggage. They have been transformed like a butterfly being released from its cocoon.

[2] *Do not conform to the pattern of this world, but be transformed by the renewing of your mind.*

Then you will be able to test and approve
what God's will is—
his good, pleasing and perfect will.

– Romans 12:2 (NIV)

These individuals are eager to learn how to take care of their body. "Healthy" and "Fit" are now their middle names. Their attitude has taken them to a higher ground. They feel strong in their bodies, minds, and spirits. Their faith has become a shield to protect them and they carry that shield everywhere.

Prayer

Dear Heavenly Father, I am thankful you are my director and you have given me hope; therefore I will press forward to a healthier me.

Activity

This new attitude helps strengthens the mind, body, and soul.

Exercise builds ups self-esteem and confidence. Exercising five times a week for thirty minutes a day can lower your weight and blood pressure and blood glucose levels, and strengthen brain cells. Exercise helps you to become more alert.

The formula for exercise is FITT:

Frequency	3 to 5 times at week
Intensity	65-85% of your target heart rate
Time	at least 30 minutes or longer
Type	aerobic dance, walking, swimming, bicycling, strength training, stretching

But don't forget to strengthen your spiritual muscles, too.

F	faith
I	intense interpersonal relationship you have with God
T	time spent with God by prayer, meditating
T	trust developed as you spend time with God

And with trust, you learn to OBEY HIM.

Exercise makes you feel good about yourself. Your confidence level rises and fear drops from your lips. Tapping the power God has given will move you forward and upward.

DAY 38
Healthy Mind = Healthy Temple

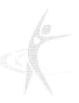

Scripture

[2] *Beloved, I pray that you may prosper in every way and [that your body] may keep well, even as [I know] your soul keeps well and prospers.*

3 JOHN 1:2 (AMP)

Devotional

You have a blueprint for keeping your body healthy. Revisit that plan, and, most of all, be flexible.

Remember these things you can do to stay healthy.

- Eat a healthy breakfast.
- Eat your meals every four to five hours apart.
- Eat at least five to seven fruits and vegetables a day.
- Drink plenty of water.
- Lower your fat, salt, and sugar intake.
- Get plenty of sleep.

- Take power naps; you will feel rejuvenated and ready for the afternoon's or evening's activities.
- Minimize your time spent watching television.
- Exercise three to five times a week.

If you do not know how to cook, check out classes at your local community college or the local kitchenware store. Or start a cooking class at church and hire a chef to come and teach the congregation. There are small culinary schools that wouldn't mind partnering with your church to offer classes. This will help their students get experience as well as your group learning how to eat healthy.

Prayer

Dear Heavenly Father, thanks for the people you sent into my life to provide instruction on learning how to take care of my temple.

DAY 39
Inside
Out

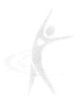

Scripture

[8] *This will bring health to your body and nourishment to your bones.*

PROVERBS 3:8 (TNIV)

Devotional

Good nutrition, exercise, and stress reduction techniques are the key elements to maintaining a healthy lifestyle. These can reduce your risk of obesity and chronic illnesses.

But *Being Fabulously Fit* is not only eating and exercising right but also living by the Word of God. *Being Fabulously Fit* is being healthy and strong from the inside out.

Don't skip breakfast, the important meal of the day. It provides you with energy, keeps you awake, and promotes brain power.

Don't skip praying in the morning. It starts your day, providing you with the energy to get you through the storms, obstacles, and hurdles of life. In the spiritual world, skipping prayer time promotes a poor relationship with God. And a poor relationship with God causes doubt, low self-esteem, lack of confidence, and lack of faith and hope.

Don't skip either one.

Believe it or not, the three key factors—good nutrition, exercise, and stress reduction techniques—can nourish your body, mind, and soul.

When you are feeling that "new attitude," it penetrates from the inside to the outside. There is a glow about you that everyone sees, and their attitudes change toward you—and themselves.

Exercise + Fitness + Faith = A New Attitude

And no one or nothing can destroy the winner in you.

Prayer

Dear Heavenly Father, my soul thirsts for your guidance and direction in providing me the right words to nourish my body, mind, and soul.

DAY 40
Winner

Scripture

⁷ *I have fought the good fight, I have finished the race, I have kept the faith.*

2 TIMOTHY 4:7 (TNIV)

Devotional

Good! Congratulations!!!!!!!!

You are a Winner and a Worshipper. I knew you would make it in keeping the faith and fighting the battle and now you have WON. Changing to a healthier lifestyle can be challenging and probably caused some tears and pain, yet you stayed on the course.

Along the way, you wanted to give in, but you didn't because of the determination and drive to honor your temple.

The journey became easier; perseverance wouldn't let go. And the fear of the unknown was knocked down by your strong faith in God. This journey took you through some valleys and roads that twisted and turned, yet your prayers were answered and you made it through.

> *. . . [I]n all your ways submit to him,*
> *and he will make your paths straight.*
>
> PROVERBS 3:6 (TNIV)

And God did.

You learned some new information about yourself; you gained strength to overcome those bad eating habits; you embraced the struggle with help, courage, and persistence to stay on the course. Endurance was dug, to help you stand the test of time.

> *Let it do its work so you become mature and*
> *well-developed, not deficient in any way.*
>
> JAMES 1:4 (MSG)

Faith became your shield to protect you from FEAR of moving forward.

> *I will trust and not be afraid*
>
> ISAIAH 12:2 (NIV)

I want to thank you for staying on the course and now *Being Fabulously Fit in God's Kingdom.*

Prayer

Dear Heavenly Father, with all the information given to me, I will give the body physical and spiritual food. I will train my temple to become healthy and fit, so I can better serve you and others.

Appendices

APPENDIX 1

Exercise Table

MON	TUES	WED	THURS	FRI	SAT	SUN
Day 1 walk treadmill sit-ups	**Day 2** biceps triceps	**Day 3** stretching	**Day 4** rest	**Day 5** walk treadmill sit-ups	**Day 6** biceps triceps	**Day 7** rest
Day 8 leg lifts sit-ups	**Day 9** walk biceps triceps	**Day 10** stretch sit-ups	**Day 11** rest	**Day 12** walk treadmill sit-ups	**Day 13** biceps triceps	**Day 14** walk leg lifts sit-ups
Day 15 walk stretching sit-ups	**Day 16** rest	**Day 17** walk biceps triceps	**Day 18** leg lifts sit-ups	**Day 19** rest	**Day 20** walk stretching sit-ups	**Day 21** biceps triceps
Day 22 leg lifts sit-ups	**Day 23** walk stretching	**Day 24** walk biceps triceps sit-ups	**Day 25** rest	**Day 26** walk leg lifts set-ups	**Day 27** biceps triceps	**Day 28** walk stretching sit-ups
Day 29 rest	**Day 30** leg lifts sit-ups	**Day 31** walk biceps triceps	**Day 32** stretching sit-ups	**Day 33** rest	**Day 34** walk leg lifts sit-ups	**Day 35** biceps triceps
Day 36 walk stretching sit-ups	**Day 37** rest	**Day 38** walk biceps triceps	**Day 39** leg lifts sit-ups	**Day 40** rest reflect renew		

APPENDIX 2
Planning Your Meals

Make healthy choices by making sure that half your plate is fruits and vegetables. Add a quarter protein and a quarter starches (breads, cereal, grains, rice, pasta) to complete the plate.

Each plate should consist of a variety of foods, textures, and colors. The darker the color, the more antioxidants. Oxidants/free radicals are particles that are released from the body when it is under stress. When you eat foods such as fruits and vegetables of various colors, their minerals and vitamins and the antioxidants fight against the free radicals that are harming your body.

Choose lean meats/cuts such as tenderloin, fish, the white meat of chicken, and poultry. And remove the skin, as that is where most of the fat is. Learn to eat other protein sources such as tofu and beans.

Limit your amount of processed foods, including luncheon meats.

It is okay to have snacks, but make sure they are a part of your calories for the day.

Buff up with bran: Grandma called it roughage. It helps to lower your weight, your blood cholesterol level, and your blood pressure.

Shake the habit: Choose to use more herbs and spices in your diet.

Bone up with calcium-rich foods: These include broccoli, low-fat milk, and other low-fat diary products.

APPENDIX 3
Cooking Tips

1. Choose lean fish, poultry, and lean cuts of meats.

2. Eat more fish, including salmon with its omega fatty acids that are good for the heart.

3. Use water-packed tuna.

4. Bake, broil, and poach your meats.

5. Limit the eggs to two a week.

6. Serve gravies and sauces on the side.

7. Choose low-fat salad dressings, and limit yourself to one tablespoon if you are using regular salad dressing.

8. Make gravy from low-fat, low-sodium broth.

9. Look for margarine made with olive oil or yogurt, such as Brummel & Brown™.

10. Instead of creams for dips, use low-fat plain yogurt.

APPENDIX 4
Healthy Snacks

- fresh fruit
- raw vegetables
- popcorn
- 100-calorie cookies
- cheese and crackers
- celery sticks with hummus or low-fat cottage cheese on top
- salsa and crackers
- fruit smoothie
- cereal and low-fat milk
- yogurt with fruit
- half a banana with one tablespoon of peanut butter
- three ounces of tuna fish with five crackers
- half a small potato with one tablespoon of salsa on top
- three graham crackers with four ounces of low-fat milk
- one ounce of trail mix

- one small apple chopped; put cinnamon on top and microwave for two minutes or until soft
- low-sodium V-8 Juice™
- apple slices topped with peanut butter

Healthy Banana Split: one banana with ¼ cup low-fat yogurt; sprinkle with oatmeal or your favorite grain cereal

Mini-Pizza: ½ English muffin with one ounce of low-fat mozzarella cheese and one to two tablespoons of tomato or pizza sauce; microwave

With packaged snacks, read the Nutrition Facts labels on the product to be sure you are following serving size.

Snack List

MON	TUES	WED	THUR	FRI	SAT	SUN
Day 1 1 oz trail mix	**Day 2** popcorn	**Day 3** 10 grapes	**Day 4** 1 oz. trail mix	**Day 5** 10 grapes	**Day 6** 1 slice of cheese 5 crackers	**Day 7** ½ cup of fruit cocktail
Day 8 3 oz. tuna fish 5 crackers	**Day 9** 1 pear 5 almonds	**Day 10** ½ cup low-fat pudding	**Day 11** sugar-free Popsicle™	**Day 12** 5 crackers 1 oz. Monterey Jack cheese	**Day 13** 6 oz. fruit smoothie	**Day 14** ½ cup soup 5 crackers
Day 15 10 grapes	**Day 16** 3 celery sticks with 1 oz. cottage cheese	**Day 17** 1 oz. Polly-O™ string cheese	**Day 18** ½ cup low-fat pudding	**Day 19** 1 oz. unsalted pretzels	**Day 20** 1 oz. peanut butter in a celery stick	**Day 21** 1 oz. turkey slice* 1 oz. ham slice*

MON	TUES	WED	THUR	FRI	SAT	SUN
Day 22 1 pear 1 slice low-fat cheese	**Day 23** 1 oz. peanut butter 1 apple	**Day 24** 1 oz. trail mix	**Day 25** 1 apple, diced**	**Day 26** 6 oz. unsalted V-8 Juice™	**Day 27** 1 oz. salsa 5 small crackers***	**Day 28** 6 oz. fruit smoothie
Day 29 5 crackers ½ cup chicken salad	**Day 30** ½ cup peaches	**Day 31** 3 graham crackers 4 oz. low-fat milk	**Day 32** ½ cup watermelon	**Day 33** 2-100 calorie cookies	**Day 34** 1 poached egg 1 slice toast	**Day 35** 1 oz. pretzels dipped into 1 tbsp. peanut butter
Day 36 ¼ cup cottage cheese ½ cup diced peaches	**Day 37** 6 oz. yogurt	**Day 38** 4 graham crackers 4 oz. low-fat milk	**Day 39** 1 small banana 10 nuts	**Day 40** 1 cup fruit salad		

* Wrap turkey and ham slices around carrots or celery sticks and dip into your favorite low-fat sauce.

** Dice apple into small pieces and sprinkle cinnamon on top; then microwave for one to two minutes or until apple becomes soft.

*** Place salsa on crackers and microwave for one minute.

APPENDIX 5:
Healthy Eating in Special Circumstances

The Holidays

- Plan ahead.
- Choose healthier versions of the foods you like.
- Remove foods early from the table to prevent overeating.
- Holidays can be emotional, so plan ahead and delegate activities when preparing foods so you will not be tempted to eat more than usual.
- Plan for relaxation time for yourself.
- Get a nap in if you feel fatigue.

Traveling

- Plan ahead.
- Call ahead to find out how the restaurant prepares the food.
- Share entrèes.

- Include walking tours, or even a bicycling tour, in your travels.
- Avoid the midnight buffet on the cruise ship.
- Sign up for the cruise ship's aerobics classes.
- Take a healthy plate with you, because then you know at least one meal is healthy.

At a Party

- Plan ahead.
- Stand with your back to the table.
- Keep both hands full, one holding a water glass and the other a small plate.
- Eat off the salad plate instead of a dinner plate, to control your portion sizes.
- Talk a lot at the party; that way you will focus on entertaining the crowd instead of on the food.
- Eat more from the salad bar.

APPENDIX 6
Questions & Answers about Fiber

What is fiber?
Fiber is the skin on plants/fruit such as apples, peaches, oranges, and pears, and "strings" in foods such as yams or celery.

There are two types of fiber:

Insoluble – cannot digest; prevents constipation— peels, seeds, kernels, strings, nuts, and beans

Soluble – dissolves in water; characterized as stickiness after cooking—beans, oats, vegetables, peas, barley

Why should we eat fiber?
* controls our weight by creating fullness; therefore you will not eat as much
* decreases risk of colon cancer
* reduces blood cholesterol levels
* reduces blood glucose levels
* prevents constipation

Where can we find fiber?

- whole grains
- breads
- cereals
- wheat bran
- fresh fruits and vegetables
- peas
- beans
- nuts
- seeds
- brown rice

How much fiber should we eat?

Eat at least 20 to 35 grams a day. Men need 38 grams; women need 25.

APPENDIX 7
Seasonings

Herbs/Spices	Ways to Use Them
Basil	eggs, fish, tomato sauce, vegetables, pastas
Bay Leaves	soups, stews, boiled beef
Caraway Seeds	roast pork, vegetables, carrots, onions, celery
Celery Powder	soups, salads, deviled eggs
Curry Powder	chicken, lamb, eggs, rice, fish
Dill	salads, chicken, fish
Fennel	pork, poultry, seafood dishes
Garlic	meats, stews, soups, salads, stir-fried vegetables
Nutmeg	apple dishes, vegetables
Onion Powder	meat, soups, stews
Oregano	Italian dishes, stews, soups
Paprika	for color, browning of roast chicken or turkey, potato salad
Pepper, Black	salads, meats, soups, stews, eggs
Pepper, Red	meat sauces, gravies, eggs, fish, vegetables, stews, chili
Rosemary	potatoes, peas, squash, stews, soups, vegetables
Sage	stuffing, poultry, pork, lamb, veal
Thyme	Italian dishes, meats, vegetables

Shopping List

Cereals
- [ ] bran flakes
- [ ] raisin bran
- [ ] cornflakes
- [ ] Cheerios™
- [ ] Special K™
- [ ] Kashi™
- [ ] oatmeal
- [ ] Fiber One™
- [ ] shredded wheat

Produce (fresh/frozen)
- [ ] apples
- [ ] bananas
- [ ] oranges
- [ ] grapefruit
- [ ] melon
- [ ] pineapples
- [ ] strawberries
- [ ] lemons
- [ ] salad greens
- [ ] onions
- [ ] potatoes
- [ ] sweet potatoes

Salad Dressing
- [ ] fat-free salad dressing
- [ ] fat-free mayonnaise
- [ ] mustard
- [ ] catsup
- [ ] taco sauce
- [ ] picante sauce
- [ ] vinegar
- [ ] balsamic vinaigrette

Breads/Grains
- [ ] whole wheat bread
- [ ] rye bread
- [ ] low-cal bread
- [ ] bagels
- [ ] pitas
- [ ] brown rice
- [ ] pasta

Meats
- [ ] chicken
- [ ] turkey
- [ ] tuna/salmon canned in water
- [ ] fresh fish

Protein
- [ ] yogurt (nonfat)
- [ ] peanut butter
- [ ] tofu
- [ ] beans
- [ ] peas
- [ ] hummus
- [ ] EggBeaters™
- [ ] eggs

Beverages

- ☐ skim milk
- ☐ 1% milk
- ☐ orange juice
- ☐ coffee/tea
- ☐ sugar-free cocoa drink

Miscellaneous

- ☐ vegetable oil
- ☐ garlic
- ☐ soy sauce
- ☐ brown sugar
- ☐ ginger, fresh or powdered
- ☐ crushed tomatoes
- ☐ tomato paste
- ☐ basil, oregano, black paper
- ☐ lemon juice
- ☐ jelly/jam
- ☐ bouillon or broth (without fat or salt)

APPENDIX 9
Walking Chart

	Miles	Minutes	Steps
Monday			
Tuesday			
Wednesday			
Thursday			
Friday			
Saturday			
Sunday			

	Miles	Minutes	Steps
Monday			
Tuesday			
Wednesday			
Thursday			
Friday			
Saturday			
Sunday			

	Miles	Minutes	Steps
Monday			
Tuesday			
Wednesday			
Thursday			
Friday			
Saturday			
Sunday			

	Miles	Minutes	Steps
Monday			
Tuesday			
Wednesday			
Thursday			
Friday			
Saturday			
Sunday			

APPENDIX 10
Target Heart Rate Chart

After a 20-30 minute aerobic workout, check your pulse for 15 seconds; then multiply the number by 4—that is your target heart rate. You want to work out in that range.

Look for your age and walk your finger across the chart to find what your heart rate should be. If you are 20 beats or more above your rate, start slowing down or reduce your intensity.

Age	Maximum Heart Rate	Target Heart Rate (Beats/Minute 60 to 80%)	10 Second Count (beats/10 seconds)
20	200	120-160	20-27
25	195	117-156	19-26
30	190	117-156	19-26
35	185	111-148	18-25
40	180	108-144	18-24
45	175	105-140	17-23
50	170	102-136	17-23
55	165	99-132	16-22
60	160	96-128	16-21
65	155	93-124	15-20

APPENDIX 11
Know Your Numbers for Spiritual Fitness

2 And be not conformed to this world: but be ye transformed by the renewing of your mind, that ye may prove what is that good, and acceptable, and perfect, will of God.

ROMANS 12:2 (KJV):

1 O God, thou art my God; early will I seek thee: my soul thirsteth for thee, my flesh longeth for thee in a dry and thirsty land, where no water is; . . .

PSALM 63:1 (KJV):

23 Jesus said unto him, If thou canst believe, all things are possible to him that believeth.

MARK 9:23 (KJV):

19 But my God shall supply all your need according to his riches in glory by Christ Jesus.

PHILIPPIANS 4:19 (KJV):

Know Your Numbers for Better Health

Cholesterol

LDL (bad)	under 100
HDL (good)	50 and above

Blood Pressure

Normal	under 120/80
High	over 140/90

Glucose

Normal	70-99
High	100 and above

Body Mass Index

Normal	18.5-24.9
Overweight	25.0-29.9
Obese	30.0-39.9
Morbidly Obese	40.0 and above

Training Hard

SUN	MON	TUE	WED	THU	FRI	SAT
walk sit-ups	biceps triceps leg lifts	rest	biceps triceps leg lifts	walk sit-ups	rest	biceps triceps leg lifts

SUN	MON	TUE	WED	THU	FRI	SAT
walk sit-ups	rest	walk sit-ups	biceps triceps leg lifts	rest	biceps triceps leg lifts	walk sit-ups

Alternative Workout

SUN	MON	TUE	WED	THU	FRI	SAT
full body*	walk	rest	full body*	walk	rest	full body*

SUN	MON	TUE	WED	THU	FRI	SAT
walk	rest	full body*	walk	rest	full body*	walk

* Biceps, triceps, sit-ups and lef lifts

Training Hard Exercises

Bicep Curls
1. Sit or stand with feet firmly on the floor.
2. Hold weights in your hands at your sides with palms facing upward.
3. Raise weights shoulder height and exhale.
4. Return to starting position and inhale.
5. Do 3 sets of 10-12 repetitions
6. Rest between sets for 1-2 minutes

Triceps kickback
1. Place your left hand on a chair for balance
2. Stand with left foot behind right foot.
3. Next raise your right hand to chest height. And inhale
4. Extend your right hand behind you and exhale.
5. Return weight back to chest.
6. Do 3 sets of 10 to 12 repetitions
7. Rest between sets for 1-2 minutes.
8. Repeat sequence with left hand.

Sit-Ups
1. Lie on floor with knees.
2. Place hands behind your head with elbows out by your ears. Inhale
3. Next curl your body forward and contract your abdominal (stomach) muscles. Exhale
4. Return to starting position.
5. Do 15-25 sit-ups per set. Resting between sets.

Leg Lifts
1. Lie on your right side on the floor.
2. Straighten your right arm on the floor or place under your head.
3.   Bend your right leg.(the leg closest to the floor)
4. Keep your left- leg straight. inhale
5. Next slowly raise your left leg halfway up and exhale.
6. Slowly return to starting position.
7. Do 2-3 sets of 10 to 12 repetitions. Rest between sets for one minute.
8. Repeat sequence on the left side.

Author

Renee Wiggins has mentored, trained, and changed lives in the health and wellness field for more than twenty years. A strong believer in, and encourager for, living an authentic healthy lifestyle, Renee specializes in designing customized lifestyle programs for individuals.

In addition, Renee conducts workshops and seminars on healthy living. Her special areas of expertise include diabetes, weight management, and stress management.

Renee is a registered and licensed dietitian, certified massage therapist, and a certified health and wellness coach.

She is also the author of several books:

Can I Exercise Sitting Down?

Stress Down and Lift UP:
Find Joy in Your Journey

Transformations: Give UP the Struggle

Renee can be reached at
renee@resultsbyrenee.com.

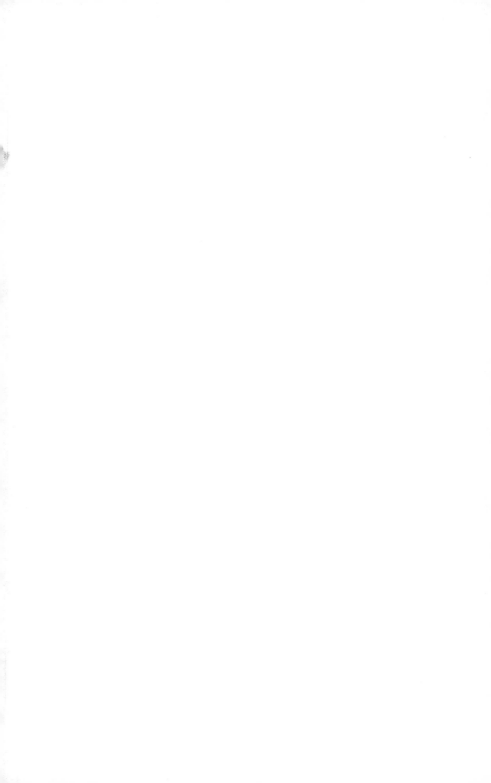

CPSIA information can be obtained at www.ICGtesting.com
Printed in the USA
BVOW08s1639071113

335456BV00001B/21/P